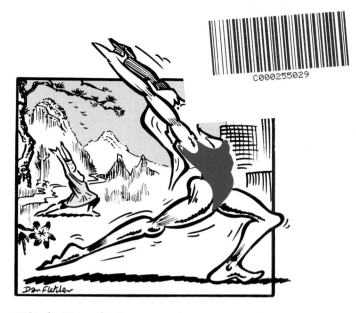

Vital Touch is a unique exercise programme deriving from the ancient Oriental art of *Do-In*. *Do-In* means literally 'self-massage' and involves the stimulation of special acupressure points.

Now available for the first time as a series of practical, easy-to-follow illustrations with notes, these exercises are simple to learn and require very little space.

Do-In can be used not only to revitalise tired muscles and low spirits but also to relieve a stiff, tense body and a stressed mind.

VITAL TOUCH

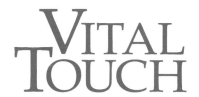

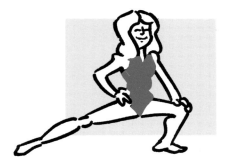

*Japanese Do-In exercises
for physical energy
and mental relaxation.*

SIMON BROWN

with illustrations by
DAN FLETCHER

A COMMUNITY HEALTH FOUNDATION PUBLICATION

VITAL TOUCH
Japanese Do-In exercises for
physical energy and mental relaxation

Published by the Community Health Foundation
188 Old Street, London EC1V 9BP.

First published 1991

© The Community Health Foundation

ISBN 0 9518443 0 X

Made and printed in Great Britain by
Helios Graphics, London SE13 5AD.
Phototypeset in Palatino.

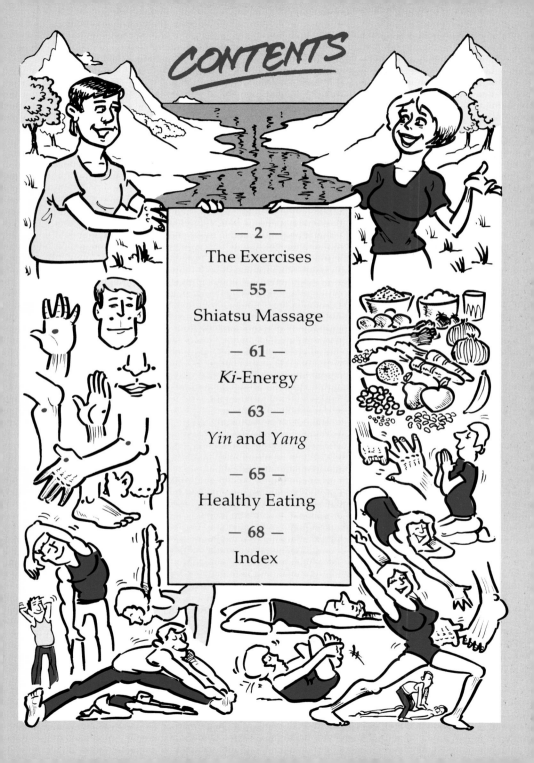

CONTENTS

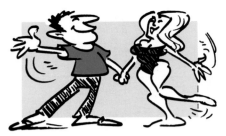

INTRODUCTION

Vital Touch is a unique exercise programme deriving from the ancient Oriental art of *Do-In*. *Do-In* literally means 'Self Massage' and combines relaxing stretches, invigorating massage and the stimulation of special acupressure points. The principles of *Do-In* originated in China about 2600 B.C. at the time of the Yellow Emperor, and were later developed and refined in Japan. *Do-In* has since evolved into a comprehensive and practical set of exercises that are easy to learn and require very little space.

A *Do-In* programme can be used not only to revitalise tired muscles and low spirits but also to relieve a stiff, tense body and a stressed mind. I have found that a morning *Do-In* session helps me feel refreshed, energetic and ready for the day, and the same routine in the evening relaxes me after a long day's work and guarantees a peaceful, deep, night's sleep.

Regular massage of the acupressure points is good for keeping in touch with the body and can prevent aches, pains and minor illnesses. Stimulating these points can often provide quick, effective relief from all kinds of discomfort.

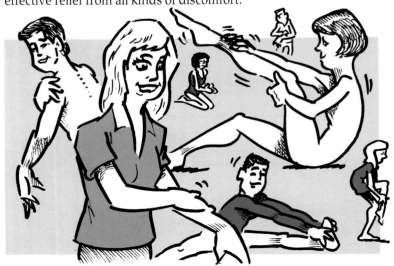

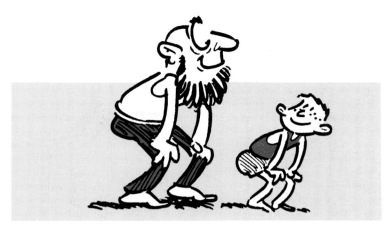

These exercises are ideal for anyone, from children to the elderly. My 3½-year-old son loves to imitate me doing *Do-In* in the morning. In his book ***Beating the Odds***, Dr Hugh Faulkner placed a great importance on these exercises in his recovery from pancreatic cancer. He still has a daily *Do-In* routine at the age of 77.

The sources for my description of the principles of *Do-In* and the acupressure points are from my many years of study with Michio Kushi, Shizuko Yamamoto, Denny Waxman, Patrick McCarty and Rik Vermuyten who have devoted their careers to the study of natural healing and Oriental medicine.

I began teaching *Do-In* in 1985, in the U.S.A. and have been practicing since 1986 at the Community Health Foundation. This book will teach you a simple effective routine that has developed over 6 years in the course of my work with hundreds of *Do-In* students.

Dan Fletcher has designed this book to help the reader learn quickly and accurately. Simply follow the pictures and read the notes for each exercise. We have provided additional information on acupressure points, and the pathways of energy known as meridians. You will also find in-depth descriptions of the principles which underlie *Do-In* practice, such as *Yin* and *Yang* and *Ki*-Energy beginning on page 61.

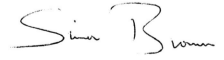

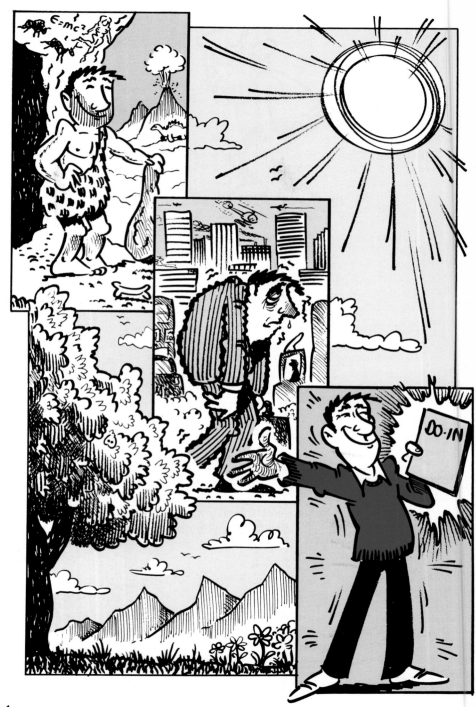

By listening to our bodies we can be more in touch with our needs, and know more exactly how to look after ourselves.

Throughout our evolution survival has always depended on strong instincts about what to eat and drink, but in modern life, many of these healthy instincts have now become dulled.

To be naturally healthy we need to listen closely and accurately to our bodies' needs so that we know when to drink because we feel thirsty and when to eat because we feel hungry. Likewise we know when to relax or sleep because our body tells us when we are tired. Our body can even tell us when to exercise and stretch our muscles.

Yet how often do we drink when we are not thirsty, eat when we are not hungry, sit around when we need to move, or overwork when we should relax?

Over the following pages we feature simple listening exercise to help "listen to your body". The idea is to know what your needs are and what makes you feel good. By focusing your mind on each part of your body you can get in touch with how each part feels. I often do this before and after *Do-In* exercise to feel what benefit that exercise has. It is also interesting to do this listening exercise before a meal and again an hour after you've eaten. See if what you ate was digestible, or if it created the feeling you wanted. You can try it before and after work or even before and after you meet a friend. See if it was a healthy experience!

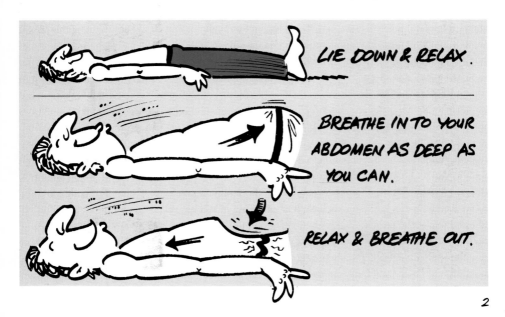

LIE DOWN & RELAX .

BREATHE IN TO YOUR ABDOMEN AS DEEP AS YOU CAN.

RELAX & BREATHE OUT.

NOW FOCUS YOUR MIND ON..

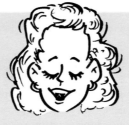

THE TOP OF YOUR HEAD - DOES IT FEEL HOT OR COLD?

YOUR BRAIN - CAN YOU STOP THE INTERNAL DIALOGUE - CAN YOU CLEAR YOUR MIND - OR IS THERE A PARTY GOING ON?

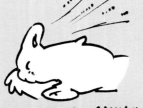

YOUR BREATH - CAN YOU FEEL IT FLOWING FREELY THROUGH YOUR NOSE?

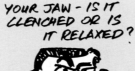

YOUR JAW - IS IT CLENCHED OR IS IT RELAXED?

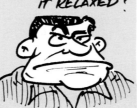

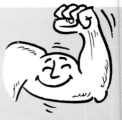

THE BACK OF YOUR HEAD - ARE THERE ANY ACHES OR PAINS?

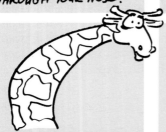

YOUR NECK - IS IT STIFF OR RELAXED?

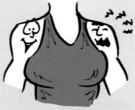

YOUR SHOULDERS ARE THEY RELAXED OR PAINFUL?

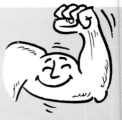

YOUR UPPER ARMS - ARE THEY TIRED OR ENERGETIC?

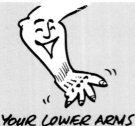

YOUR LOWER ARMS ARE THEY HEAVY OR LIGHT?

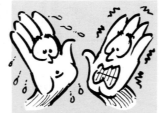

YOUR HANDS - ARE THEY HOT COLD DRY OR DAMP?

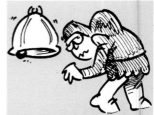

YOUR UPPER BACK - ARE THERE ANY ACHES OR PAINS

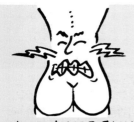

YOUR LOWER BACK IS THERE ANY TENSION?

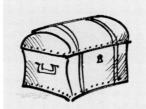

YOUR CHEST - IS YOUR BREATHING FREE AND EASY OR RESTRICTED?

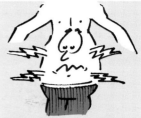

YOUR STOMACH - IS IT BLOATED - RELAXED OR NERVOUS?

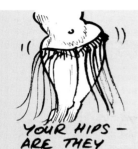

YOUR HIPS - ARE THEY RELAXED?

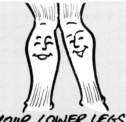

YOUR BUTTOCKS - DO THEY FEEL RELAXED?

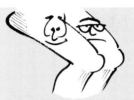

YOUR UPPER LEGS - ARE THEY TIRED OR ENERGETIC?

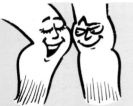

YOUR KNEES - ARE THEY STIFF - IS THERE PAIN?

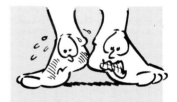

YOUR LOWER LEGS ARE THEY HEAVY OR LIGHT?

YOUR FEET - ARE THEY HOT, COLD, DAMP, OR DRY?

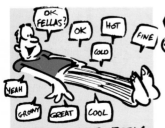

YOUR WHOLE BODY HOW DO YOU FEEL ALL OVER?

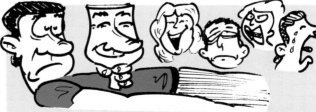

YOUR EMOTIONS - HOW DO YOU FEEL INSIDE - DO YOU FEEL HAPPY - SAD - WORRIED, CALM, DEPRESSED, POSITIVE?

LOOSEN UP

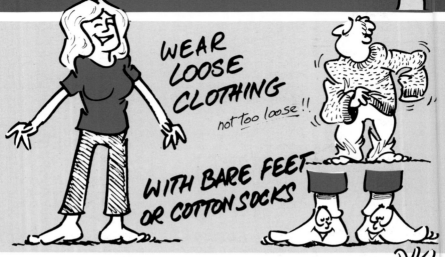

WEAR
LOOSE
CLOTHING

not too loose!!

WITH BARE FEET
OR COTTON SOCKS

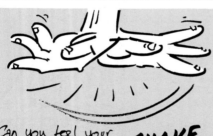

Can you feel your
blood reach the tips
of your fingers?

**SHAKE
HANDS**

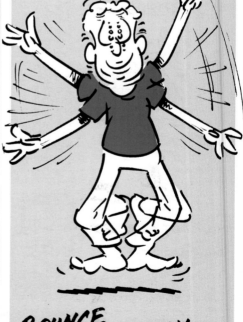

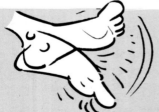

Is blood
reaching down
to your toes?

**SHAKE
FEET**

**BOUNCE
UP & DOWN**

5

SIDE TO SIDE

½ MIN

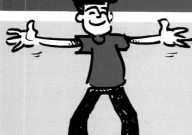

STANDING WITH LEGS SHOULDER WIDTH APART & KNEES SLIGHTLY BENT...

SWING ROUND FROM HIPS LETTING YOUR ARMS FLOP AROUND BODY TO THE LEFT - LOOKING BEHIND YOU AS FAR AS YOU CAN...

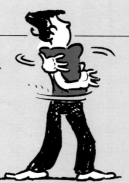

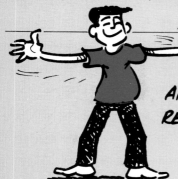

AND THEN SWING BACK KEEPING RELAXED AND FLOPPY...

ALL THE WAY ROUND TO THE RIGHT SIDE - REPEAT × 10.

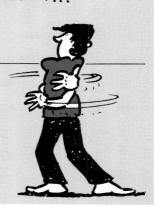

If your hip joints are painful as you turn pivot your left foot as you turn left. etc...

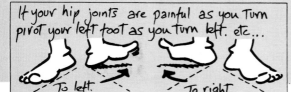

To left.   To right

6

40 SECS

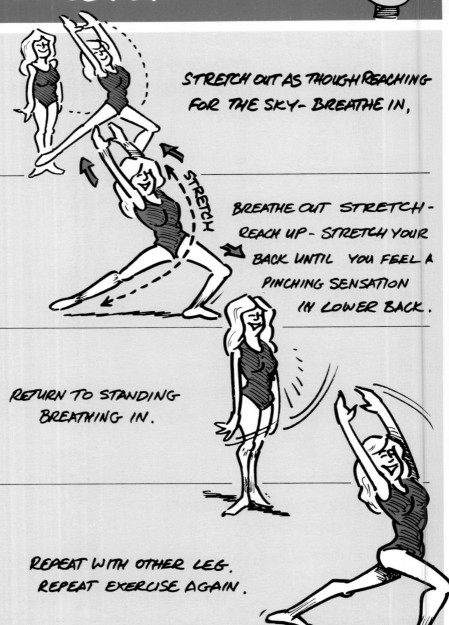

STRETCH OUT AS THOUGH REACHING FOR THE SKY - BREATHE IN,

STRETCH

BREATHE OUT STRETCH - REACH UP - STRETCH YOUR BACK UNTIL YOU FEEL A PINCHING SENSATION IN LOWER BACK.

RETURN TO STANDING BREATHING IN.

REPEAT WITH OTHER LEG. REPEAT EXERCISE AGAIN.

WINDMILL ARMS

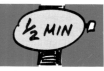

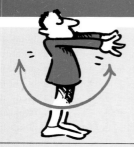

SWING YOUR ARMS BACKWARDS & FORWARDS...

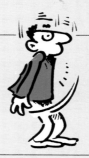

BENDING YOUR KNEES AS YOUR ARMS GO DOWN

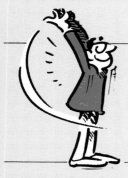

STRAIGHTEN YOUR LEGS AS YOUR ARMS GO UP

REPEAT UNTIL YOU HAVE A GOOD SWINGING MOTION WITHOUT USING SHOULDER OR ARM MUSCLES.

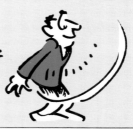

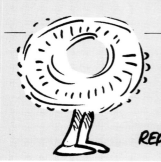

AND THEN GO INTO FULL ARM ROTATION USING BODY TO SWING ONE ARM

REPEAT WITH OTHER ARM

SHOULDER-BODY STRETCH

40 SECS

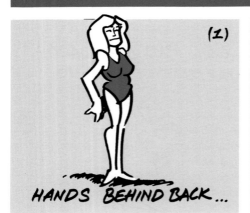

(1)

HANDS BEHIND BACK...

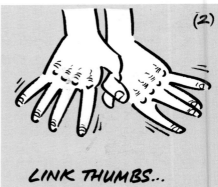

(2)

LINK THUMBS...

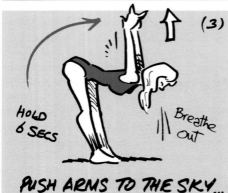

(3)

HOLD 6 SECS

Breathe Out

PUSH ARMS TO THE SKY...

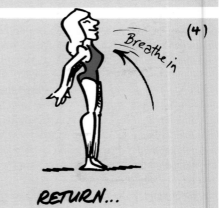

(4)

Breathe in

RETURN...

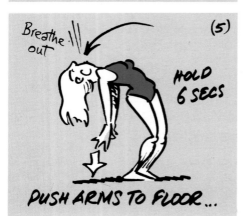

(5)

Breathe out

HOLD 6 SECS

PUSH ARMS TO FLOOR...

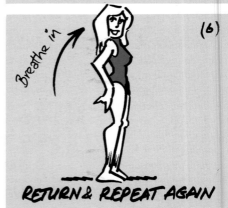

(6)

Breathe in

RETURN & REPEAT AGAIN

HAND DO-IN

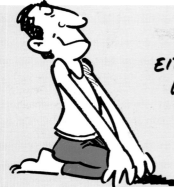

EITHER SIT OR KNEEL,
WHICHEVER IS MORE
COMFORTABLE - KNEELING
IS PREFERABLE.

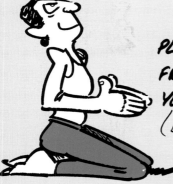

PLACE HANDS TOGETHER IN
FRONT OF NAVEL. IN THIS POSITION
YOU HAVE THE GREATEST STRENGTH.
(Experiment on lid
of tight jar)

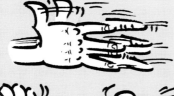

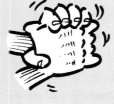

RUB HANDS VIGOROUSLY
ALL OVER.

10

RUBBING HAND & ARM TSUBOS

raditional oriental medicine describes a subtle 'life-energy' termed *Ki* or *Chi* –which flows through the organism along invisible pathways known as meridans (see *'Ki-Energy'* page 61). The acupressure points are found along each meridian where this flow of energy can be enhanced most easily. In Japan they are called *Tsubos*, and meridian charts describe 360 such points on the human body.

These principles are still used in *Do-In, Shiatsu* and acupuncture, where each point has a specific purpose and is used for specific health problems. In addition these points are used by some doctors for pain relief as massaging the points releases endorphins which function as pain killers. In China they are even used during surgery as a replacement for anaesthetics. Patrick McCarty, a shiatsu practitioner who studied acupuncture in China tells of observing brain surgery being performed in a Chinese hospital where the patient underwent surgery involving cutting through the skull. Instead of anaesthetic the patient simply had two acupuncture needles in his arm. He was awake and fully conscious throughout the whole operation.

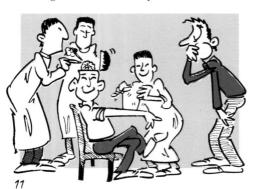

The illustrations show the location of each acupressure point with tips on how to find them. You will probably know if you have found the point, as they are often more sensitive when pressed deeply. They may feel sore, or you may feel a sharp pain or a tingling sensation. I suggest you follow the instructions and then move your thumb around slightly until you feel the greatest effect. Once you have found the point I recommend that each point is lightly massaged as you breathe in and then pressed as you breathe out. At the same time try to imagine you are breathing energy into your body as you breathe in, and into the acupressure point, on the out breath. This is shown on page 16. You can press each point as deeply as it feels good to you. Like a big stretch, you might find the pressure a little uncomfortable but it should feel as though it is doing you some good. The time taken to press each point is one long out breath, typically five seconds. Generally any one point can be pressed three times. However, a particularly sensitive point may need extra attention.

Acupressure points are often used for diagnosis. If you feel an unpleasant, sickening pain, it is often a sign that you need to improve the condition of the related organ. For example, if a point on the large intestine meridian feels un-usually sore you could try improving your diet for a while and see if it gets better.

Sometimes a point that initially feels sore will improve simply by pressing it, or you will notice it feels better after a *Do-In* session. This is another way you can keep in touch with your own body.

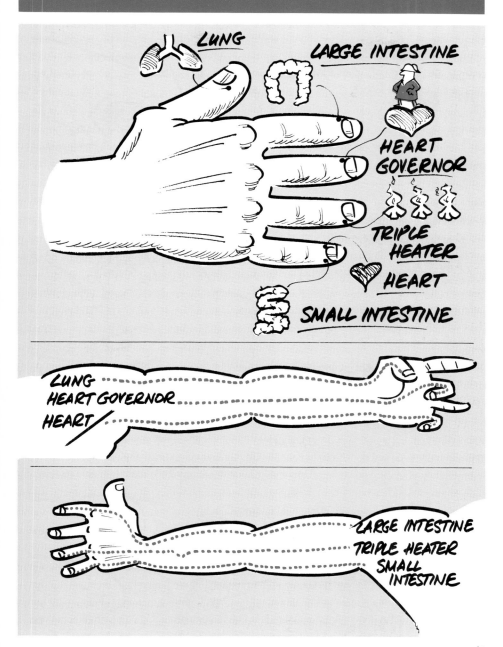

FINGER DO-IN

HOLD SIDES OF FINGER
AT BASE...

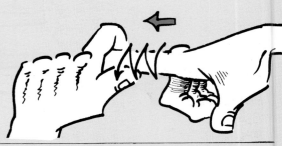

TWIST AND PULL
RUBBING ALONG
FINGER.

SQUEEZE EITHER SIDE
OF BASE OF NAIL...
(These are beginning & ends
of meridians in hands)

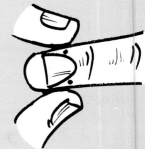

ROTATE FINGER
VIGOROUSLY.

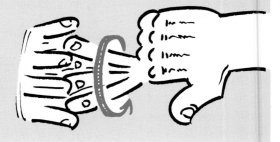

BREATHING OUT—
PULL AWAY
SHARPLY...

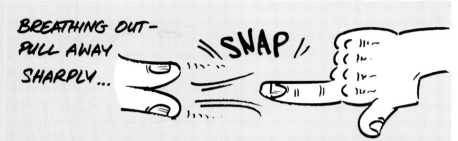

SNAP

IMAGINE EXTENDING YOUR KI
ENERGY OUT-
WARDS FROM
FINGER.

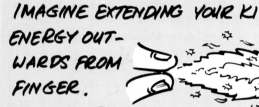

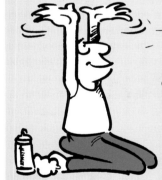

AFTER HAVING DONE ALL FINGERS
& THUMBS — SHAKE YOUR HANDS
ABOVE HEAD — IMAGINE POLISHING
THE SKY !

In Chinese medicine the tips of fingers
& toes are the most peripheral
part of body & stimulate or relax
deep inside the torso.

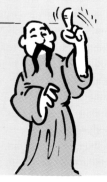

BREATHING

We are more dependent on breathing than on any other bodily function for life. If we do not breathe for 7 minutes we die. Yet breathing is something we usually pay very little attention to. Like everything else, the respiratory system needs to be exercised and kept fit. One exercise is to see how much air you can breathe in and then try to fully empty your lungs. As you first breathe in, push the air down, as though going into your abdomen. Then continue to fill the chest and finally raise your arms up and back to completely fill yourself with air. As you breathe out tighten the muscles in the abdomen to squeeze out as much air as you can.

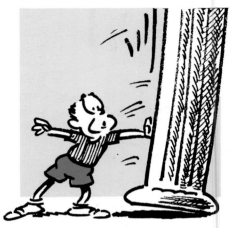

Students of the martial arts are advised to "breathe from the abdomen", which means trying to breathe so that the abdomen expands with the in breath and contracts with the out breath. This helps to massage the internal organs and increases your breathing capacity. In addition, martial arts practitioners find that such exercises have the effect of lowering the centre of gravity and increasing inner strength.

For example, try breathing out as you lift something heavy, or as you push open a spring door and you will find doing so on the out breath makes the action seem easier. In shiatsu massage, practitioners often notice that as the patient breathes out, their body also relaxes more and it is possible to stretch them further.

Try breathing out every time you exert yourself or stretch and see for yourself. After a while you may find it becomes second nature.

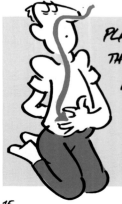

PLACE ONE HAND OVER NAVEL AND THE OTHER HAND BEHIND YOUR BACK FEEL YOUR ABDOMEN EXPAND AS YOU BREATHE IN. AS YOU BREATHE OUT CONTRACT ABDOMEN AND FEEL HANDS COME TOGETHER.

CULTIVATING KI ENERGY

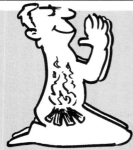

WITH AN EMPTY MIND IMAGINE A FIRE ROARING IN YOUR ABDOMEN AND AS YOU BREATHE IN - THE FLAMES ARE FANNED.

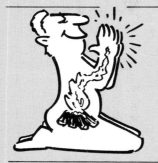

AS YOU BREATHE OUT - CONTRACTING YOUR ABDOMEN - IMAGINE FLAMES GOING UP & INTO YOUR HANDS REPEAT 6 TIMES.

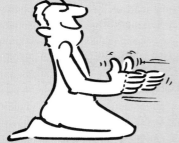

PLACE HANDS INFRONT OF NAVEL & RUB THEM TOGETHER VIGOROUSLY.

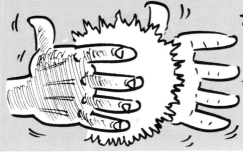

THEN PLACE YOUR HANDS 10-20 CM APART & TRY TO FEEL THE ENERGY FROM YOUR HANDS. KEEP MOVING HANDS TOGETHER AND APART- BE SENSITIVE.

PRESSING HAND & ARM TSUBOS

6 MINS

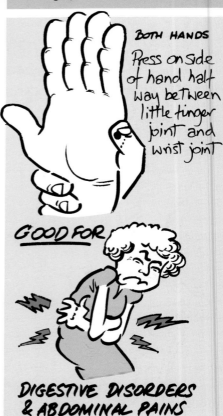

PRESS 5 SECS – 3 TIMES
SMALL INTESTINE Nº 3
"Rear Groove"

BOTH HANDS

Press on side of hand half way between little finger joint and wrist joint

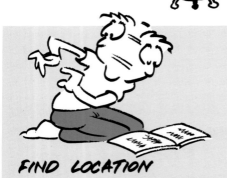

FIND LOCATION

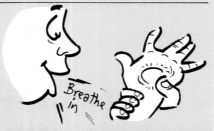

Breathe In

RUB ON & AROUND POINT FIRMLY AS YOU BREATHE IN

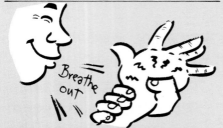

Breathe Out

PRESS HARD AND EXHALE BREATHING ENERGY INTO POINT.

GOOD FOR

DIGESTIVE DISORDERS & ABDOMINAL PAINS

SMALL INTESTINE MERIDIAN : (YANG)

Associated with absorbtion of food & taking things in. When flowing well provides feeling of contentment.

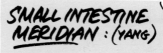

17

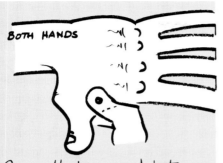

BOTH HANDS

Press fleshy mound between thumb and first finger

GOOD FOR:

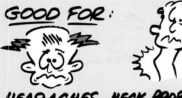

HEADACHES   **NECK PROBLEMS**

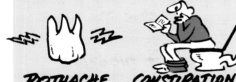

TOOTHACHE   **CONSTIPATION**

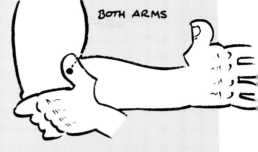

BOTH ARMS

Press at end of crease in elbow when arm bent at right angles

GOOD FOR:

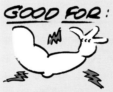 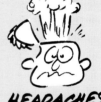

ARM PAINS   **HEADACHES**

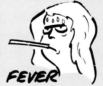 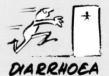

FEVER   **DIARRHOEA**

LARGE INTESTINE MERIDIAN (YANG)

Responsible for the elimination of solid waste and re-absorption of liquids. The KI energy in this meridian is good for keeping things unstuck and moving. When this energy does not flow well people often become withdrawn.

18

BOTH WRISTS

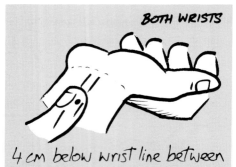

4 cm below wrist line between Two Tendons.

BOTH HANDS

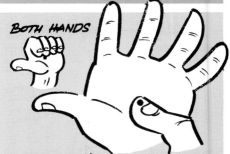

In middle of palm below middle finger when fingers clenched

GOOD FOR:

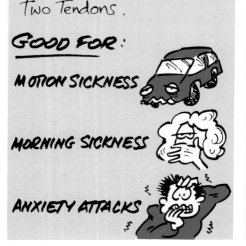

MOTION SICKNESS

MORNING SICKNESS

ANXIETY ATTACKS

GOOD FOR:

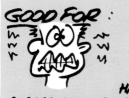

STRESS RELIEF

HASTEN END OF COLDS

OVERWORK

TONIFICATION

HEART GOVERNOR MERIDIAN (YIN)

Although there is no such organ this energy is instrumental in blood circulation. Enhancing this flow of energy creates a calming feeling. Good for stress relief.

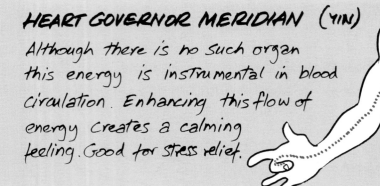

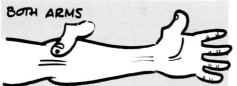

BOTH ARMS

Open arm straight out. Point just below elbow crease. Squeeze fore arm muscle.

GOOD FOR :

SORE THROATS

COUGHS

COLDS

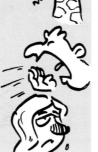

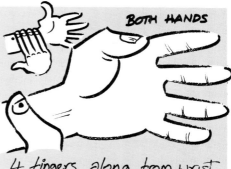

BOTH HANDS

4 fingers along from wrist on inside top of arm.

GOOD FOR :

COUGHING

ASTHMA

COLDS

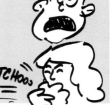

ATCHOO,,,

LUNG MERIDIAN (YIN)

Responsible for absorption of oxygen and elimination of carbon monoxide. Also influential in our ability to take in ki energy. Good for positive thinking & physical endurance When this energy is weak it becomes easier to feel depressed.

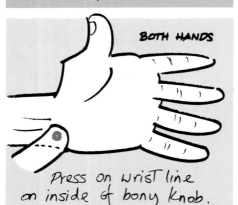

BOTH HANDS

Press on wrist line on inside of bony knob.

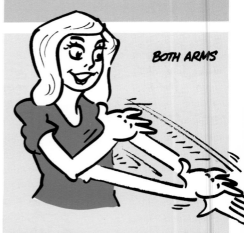

BOTH ARMS

GOOD FOR:

HYSTERIA

INSOMNIA

IRRITABILITY

GOOD FOR:

CREATING A FEELING OF WARMTH.

FROZEN SHOULDER

HEART MERIDIAN (YIN)

This energy is seen as our Spirit of Adventure providing a sense of rhythm. When imbalanced creates a feeling of hysteria and panic.

TRIPLE HEATER MERIDIAN (YANG)

3 areas on front of the torso where energy is created from food, water, & air, creates warmth and energy.

HEAD & FACE MASSAGE

 2 MINS

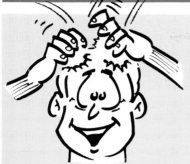

TAP TOP OF HEAD WITH FINGERS.

RUB FOREHEAD FROM SIDE TO SIDE 5 TIMES.

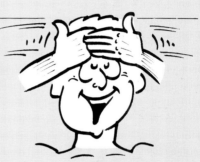

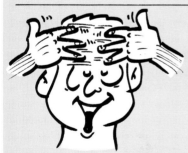

STRETCH OUTWARDS FROM CENTRE TO TEMPLES.

RUB IN CIRCULAR MOTION IN & AROUND TEMPLES - SQUEEZE OUT TENSION. THIS CAN PREVENT & RELIEVE HEADACHES.

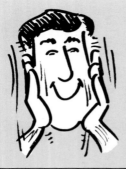

RUB CHEEKS UP & DOWN VIGOROUSLY - GOOD FOR WAKING UP & INCREASING YOUR ENERGY !

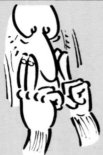

AND THE SIDES OF NOSE .

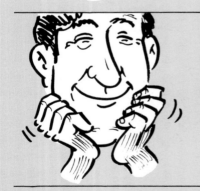

SQUEEZE ALONG JAW BONE. GOOD FOR RELAXATION AND STIMULATING SALIVA GLANDS.

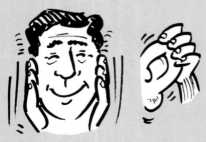

RUB EARS UP AND DOWN, THEN MASSAGE EAR & PULL GENTLY. In Chinese medicine large ears with good lobes are a sign of a strong constitution. Look at old down & outs who manage to abuse their bodies & survive.

NECK STRETCHING

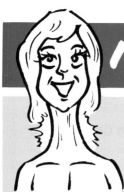

THESE EXERCISES ARE TO BE
DONE SLOWLY & CAREFULLY
- DO NOT JAR NECK!

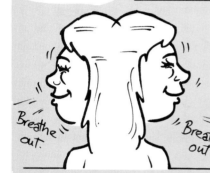

Breathe out.

Breathe out

TURN SLOWLY TO EACH
SIDE - LOOKING OVER
SHOULDER - BREATHING OUT
AT EACH STRETCH.

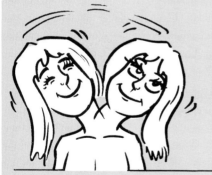

STRETCH TO EACH SIDE
BREATHING OUT.

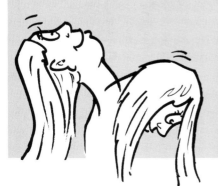

STRETCH HEAD BACKWARDS
AND FORWARDS - BREATHE
OUT AT EACH STRETCH.

24

RUBBING FACE AND HEAD TSUBOS

1 MIN

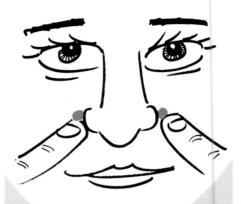

PRESS INDEX FINGERS INTO CORNERS OF NOSE & FEEL HOLLOW GROOVE.

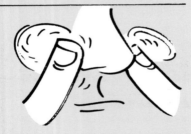

FIND LOCATION...

RUB POINT BREATHING IN...

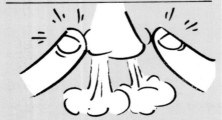

PRESS POINT BREATHING OUT FOR 5 SECS.

GOOD FOR:

NASAL OBSTRUCTIONS

CLEARING AIR PASSAGES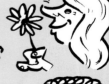

FACIAL TENSION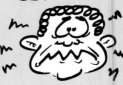

25

IF YOU HAVE BEEN KNEELING
YOU MAY BE FEELING PAIN, OR PINS
& NEEDLES IN KNEES & ANKLES!!
GET UP SLOWLY

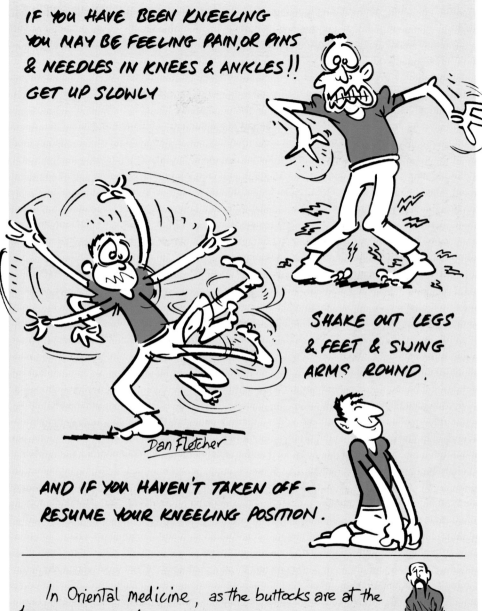

Dan Fletcher

SHAKE OUT LEGS
& FEET & SWING
ARMS ROUND.

AND IF YOU HAVEN'T TAKEN OFF -
RESUME YOUR KNEELING POSITION.

In Oriental medicine, as the buttocks are at the
opposite end of spine to head, they say pounding
buttocks stimulates the brain. Try it next time you're feeling dull.

ABDOMINAL MASSAGE

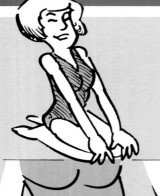

KNEEL.

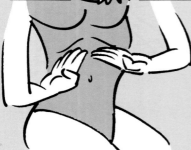

POSITION HANDS BELOW YOUR
RIBS - CLOSE TO EACH OTHER
BREATHE IN & THEN...

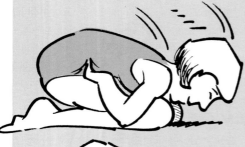

BREATH OUT AS YOU BEND
DOWN SLOWLY - GENTLY
PUSHING FINGERS UP AND
UNDER RIBS TO THE
FIRST FINGER JOINT.

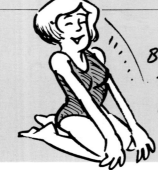

BREATHE IN AS YOU SIT UP AGAIN.
THIS EXERCISE MASSAGES
LIVER ON LEFT & STOMACH ON RIGHT

45 SECS

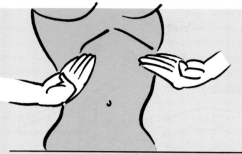

MOVE HANDS FURTHER
APART THIS TIME.

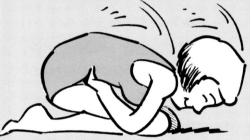

BREATHE OUT AS YOU BEND,
PRESSING LIVER ON LEFT
& PANCREAS ON RIGHT.

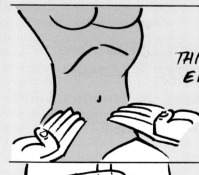

THIS TIME PLACE HANDS BELOW &
EITHER SIDE OF NAVEL PRESSING
LARGE INTESTINE. BEND
FORWARDS AS BEFORE.

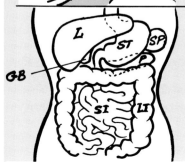

LIVER
GALL BLADDER
STOMACH
SPLEEN
PANCREAS
SMALL INTESTINE
LARGE INTESTINE

34

ABDOMINAL MASSAGE

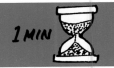 1 MIN

LIE DOWN ON BACK WITH KNEES UP...

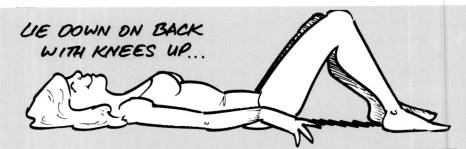

RUB ABDOMEN IN CLOCKWISE DIRECTION PRESSING FIRMLY — THIS IS THE DIRECTION FOOD PASSES THROUGH THE LARGE INTESTINE

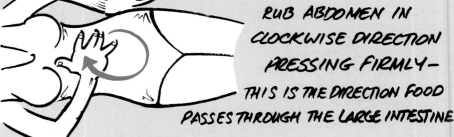

PRESS POINTS AROUND OUTER ABDOMEN PRESSING LARGE INTESTINE GOOD FOR CONSTIPATION.

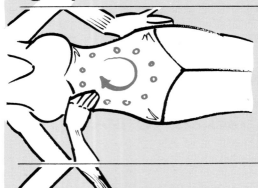

PRESSING POINTS FURTHER IN AROUND YOUR NAVEL FOR THE SMALL INTESTINE

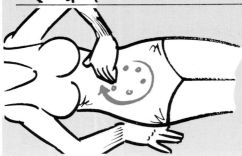

KNEE & HIP ROTATION

30 SECS

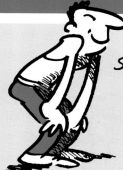

STANDING FEET TOGETHER
PLACE HANDS ON BENT KNEES...

ROTATE KNEES IN CIRCULAR MOTION...

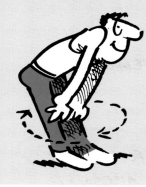

STRAIGHTENING LEGS AS THEY
GO ROUND AT BACK
REPEAT x 7 IN BOTH DIRECTIONS.

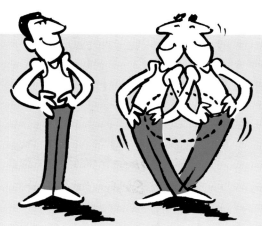

FEET TOGETHER -
ROTATE HIPS SLOWLY
STRETCHING ALL WAY
ROUND. REPEAT x 3
IN BOTH DIRECTIONS.

STANDING STRETCHES

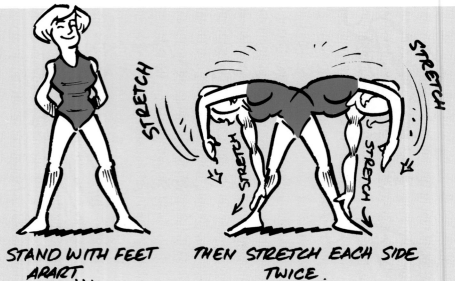

STAND WITH FEET APART...

THEN STRETCH EACH SIDE TWICE.

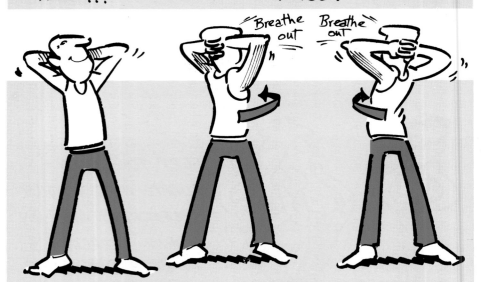

TWIST BODY ROUND SLOWLY AS FAR AS YOU CAN AND HOLD 3 SECS.

MORE...

40 SECS

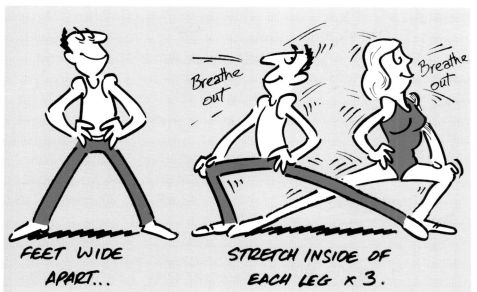

FEET WIDE APART...

STRETCH INSIDE OF EACH LEG x 3.

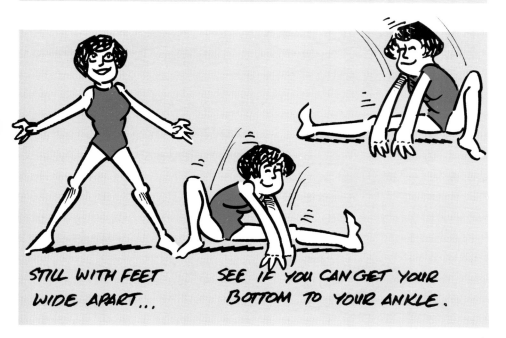

STILL WITH FEET WIDE APART...

SEE IF YOU CAN GET YOUR BOTTOM TO YOUR ANKLE.

½ MIN

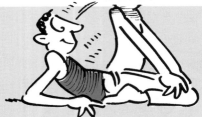

USING ELBOWS, LEAN BACK...

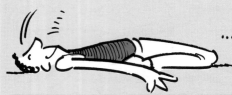

... TO LYING DOWN. BACK FLAT ON FLOOR.

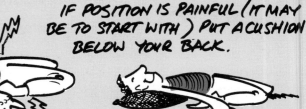

IF POSITION IS PAINFUL (IT MAY BE TO START WITH) PUT A CUSHION BELOW YOUR BACK.

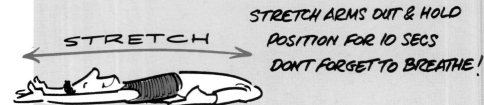

STRETCH

STRETCH ARMS OUT & HOLD POSITION FOR 10 SECS DON'T FORGET TO BREATHE!

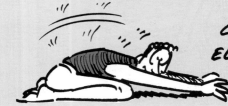

COME UP SLOWLY USING ELBOWS & STRETCH FORWARD.

1 MIN

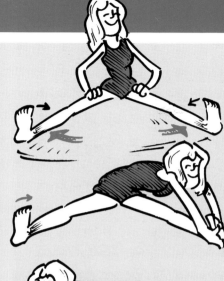

STRETCH LEGS APART AS WIDE AS POSSIBLE.

STRETCH DOWN BREATHING OUT AND HOLD TOES OR ANKLES. BREATHE IN & STRETCH BREATHING OUT.

REPEAT REMEMBERING TO KEEP TOES TOWARDS HEAD.

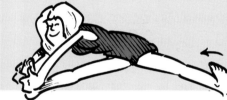

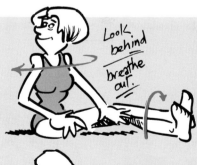

Look behind breathe out.

LEFT LEG OVER RIGHT, TWIST TO RIGHT LOOKING BACK AS FAR AS YOU CAN — USE HANDS TO PUSH YOURSELF.

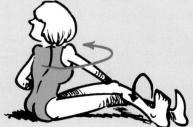

REPEAT OTHER SIDE. GOOD FOR TIGHTNESS & TENSION IN LOWER BACK.

STRETCHING & ROCKING

 1 MIN

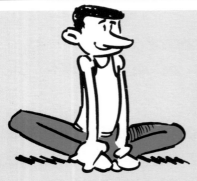

PLACE FEET TOGETHER
AND GRASP THEM...

AND USE ELBOWS TO PUSH KNEES
DOWN TOWARDS FLOOR BREATHING
OUT x 3

MOST CHILDREN CAN PUSH THEIR
KNEES DOWN TO THE GROUND.
AS ADULTS WE LOSE OUR FLEXIBILITY
BUT WITH EXERCISE WE CAN REGAIN IT.

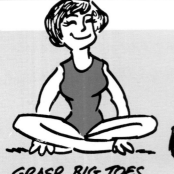 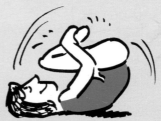 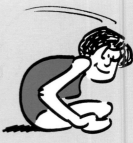

GRASP BIG TOES,
CURVE BACK AND ROLL BACKWARDS AND FORWARDS x6.
THIS EXERCISE IS GOOD FOR SPINE AS YOU ROLL ON EACH VERTEBRAE

FURTHER STRETCHES

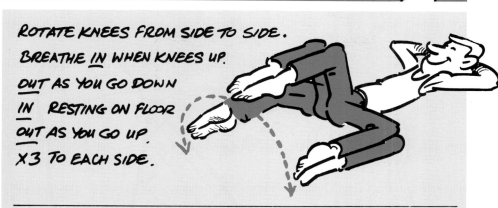

ROTATE KNEES FROM SIDE TO SIDE.
BREATHE *IN* WHEN KNEES UP.
OUT AS YOU GO DOWN
IN RESTING ON FLOOR
OUT AS YOU GO UP.
X3 TO EACH SIDE.

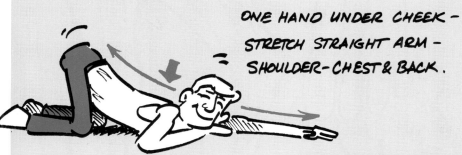

ONE HAND UNDER CHEEK –
STRETCH STRAIGHT ARM –
SHOULDER – CHEST & BACK.

REPEAT OTHER ARM.

KEEP ELBOWS TOGETHER

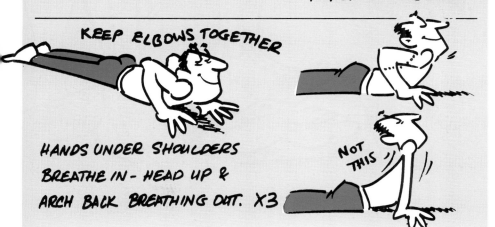

HANDS UNDER SHOULDERS
BREATHE IN – HEAD UP &
ARCH BACK BREATHING OUT. X3

NOT THIS

42

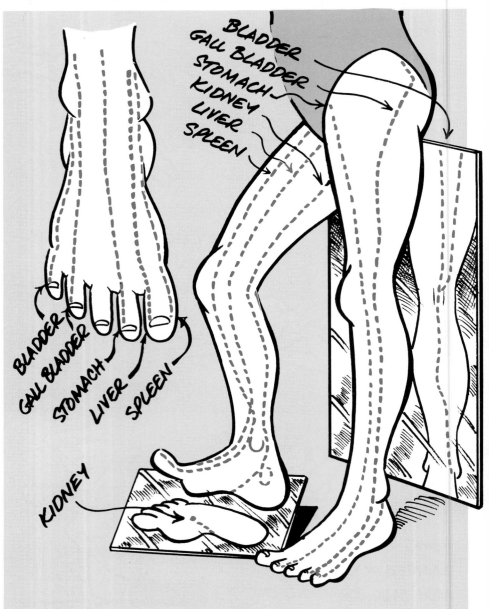

BLADDER
GALL BLADDER
STOMACH
KIDNEY
LIVER
SPLEEN

BLADDER
GALL BLADDER
STOMACH
LIVER
SPLEEN

KIDNEY

LEG POUNDING

2 MINS

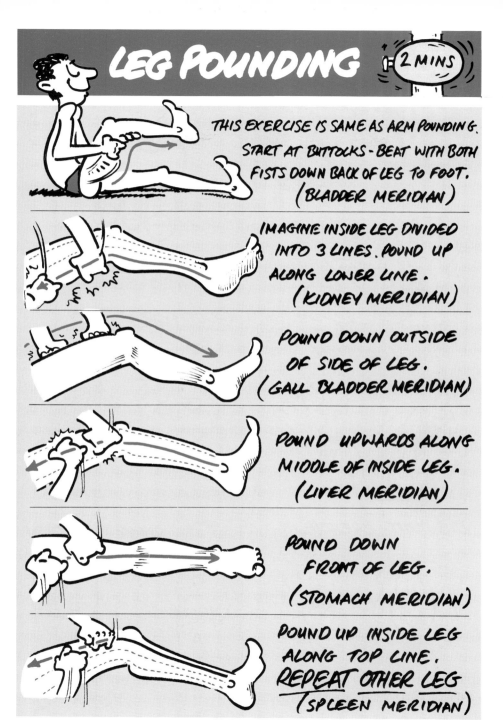

THIS EXERCISE IS SAME AS ARM POUNDING.
START AT BUTTOCKS - BEAT WITH BOTH
FISTS DOWN BACK OF LEG TO FOOT.
(BLADDER MERIDIAN)

IMAGINE INSIDE LEG DIVIDED
INTO 3 LINES. POUND UP
ALONG LOWER LINE.
(KIDNEY MERIDIAN)

POUND DOWN OUTSIDE
OF SIDE OF LEG.
(GALL BLADDER MERIDIAN)

POUND UPWARDS ALONG
MIDDLE OF INSIDE LEG.
(LIVER MERIDIAN)

POUND DOWN
FRONT OF LEG.
(STOMACH MERIDIAN)

POUND UP INSIDE LEG
ALONG TOP LINE.
REPEAT OTHER LEG
(SPLEEN MERIDIAN)

44

PRESSING FOOT & LEG TSUBOS

5 MINS

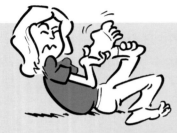

FIND LOCATION

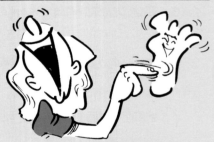

RUB POINT - BREATHE IN

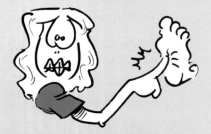

PRESS POINT - BREATHE OUT

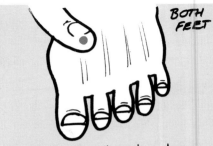

BOTH FEET

4 fingers up from bridge between big toe & 2nd toe

GOOD FOR:

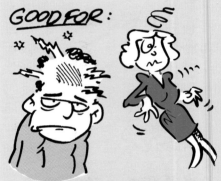

HEADACHES   DIZZINESS

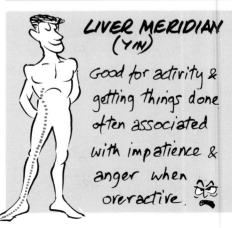

LIVER MERIDIAN (YIN)

Good for activity & getting things done often associated with impatience & anger when overactive.

45

BOTH FEET

BOTH FEET

½ way between tip of anklebone ơ Achilles Tendon

Inside foot

⅓ of way down foot from middle toe - ½ way across foot.

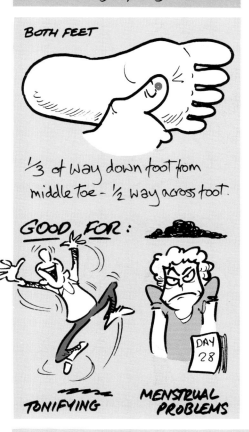

GOOD FOR:

TONIFYING

MENSTRUAL PROBLEMS

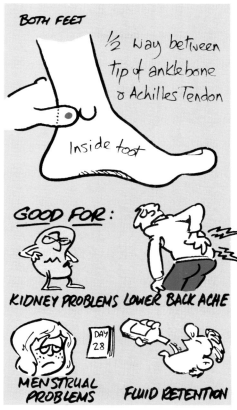

GOOD FOR:

KIDNEY PROBLEMS   LOWER BACK ACHE

MENSTRUAL PROBLEMS

FLUID RETENTION

DAY 28

KIDNEY MERIDIAN (YANG)

Responsible for fluid balance, blood quality and elimination of waste from the blood This meridian is good for confidence, vitality, and health of reproductive organs An imbalance can create feelings of fear and anxiety.

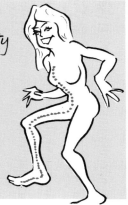

46

PRESS 5 SECS 3 TIMES
SPLEEN Nº 6
"Meeting place of 3 yin meridians"

PRESS 5 SECS 3 TIMES
BLADDER Nº 57
"In the mountain"

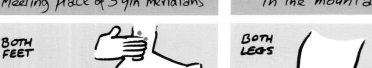

BOTH FEET

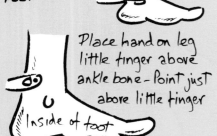

Place hand on leg little finger above ankle bone - Point just above little finger

Inside of foot

☼ Not to be used on Pregnant Women

GOOD FOR:

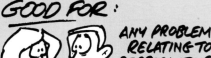

ANY PROBLEM RELATING TO REPRODUCTIVE ORGANS

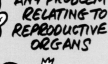

CHILD BIRTH

DIGESTIVE PROBLEMS

BOTH LEGS

In the top of the groove at beginning of the calf muscle

GOOD FOR:

MUSCLE SPASM   SCIATICA

TIRED LEGS   LOWER BACK PAIN

SPLEEN MERIDIAN
— (YIN) —

Cleanliness, order
Stability, decisiveness.
When imbalanced
can cause mood
swings, self-pity
lack of direction

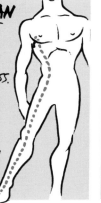

BLADDER MERIDIAN
— (YANG) —

Good for memory,
quality of fluids
which makes up 70%
of our body. Imbalance
causes insecurities
about the past.

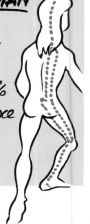

PRESS 5 SECS 3 TIMES
GALL BLADDER Nº 34
"Life Tomb spring"

PRESS 5 SECS 3 TIMES
STOMACH Nº 36
"3 miles point"

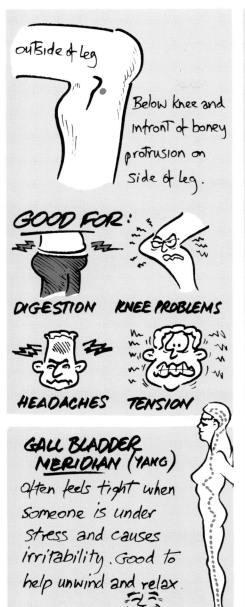

outside of leg

Below knee and infront of boney protrusion on side of leg.

GOOD FOR:

DIGESTION   **KNEE PROBLEMS**

HEADACHES   **TENSION**

GALL BLADDER MERIDIAN (YANG)

Often feels tight when someone is under stress and causes irritability. Good to help unwind and relax.

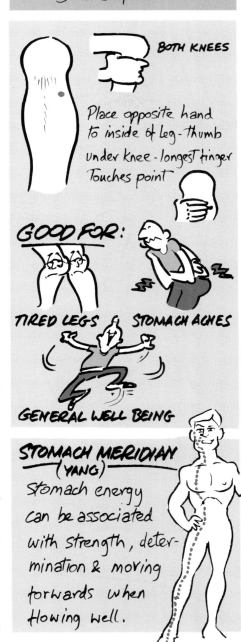

BOTH KNEES

Place opposite hand to inside of leg - thumb under knee - longest finger touches point

GOOD FOR:

TIRED LEGS   **STOMACH ACHES**

GENERAL WELL BEING

STOMACH MERIDIAN (YANG)

Stomach energy can be associated with strength, determination & moving forwards when flowing well.

48

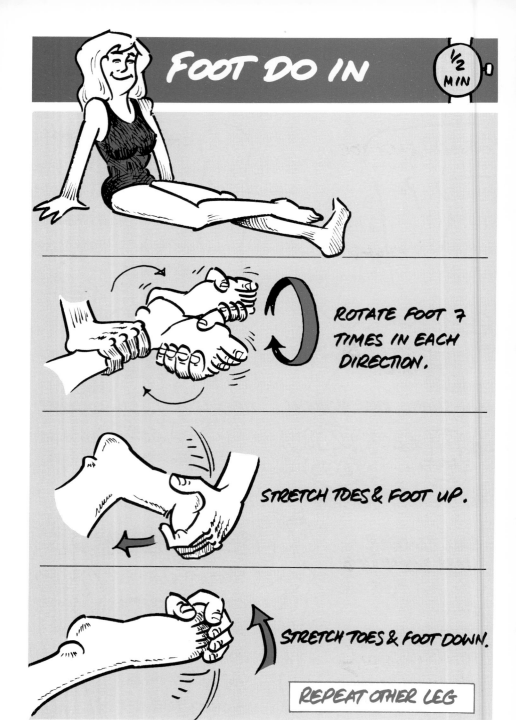

FOOT DO IN

½ MIN

ROTATE FOOT 7 TIMES IN EACH DIRECTION.

STRETCH TOES & FOOT UP.

STRETCH TOES & FOOT DOWN.

REPEAT OTHER LEG

TOE DO-IN

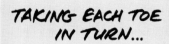 **1 MIN**

TAKING EACH TOE
IN TURN...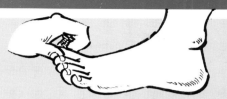

TWIST & PULL.

SQUEEZE AT BASE
OF NAIL...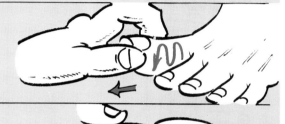

ROTATE...

PULL & BREATHE OUT.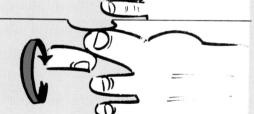
SNAP

IMAGINE EXTENDING
YOUR KI ENERGY.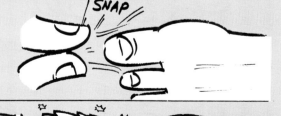

REPEAT OTHER FOOT

LAST FOOT DO-IN

1 MIN 20 SECS

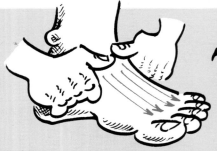

PRESS BETWEEN TENDONS ON TOP OF FOOT.

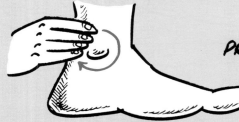

PRESS & RUB AROUND ANKLE BONE.

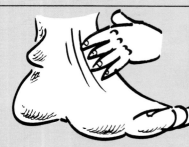

PRESS BETWEEN TENDONS ON ANKLE.

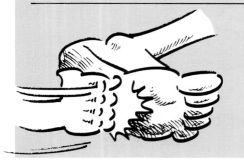

POUND SOLE.

REPEAT OTHER FOOT

FINISHING OFF

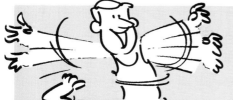

SHAKE ALL OVER...

LIKE A WET DOG!

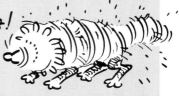

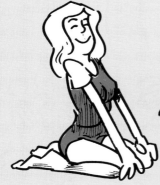

REPEAT
"LISTENING TO YOUR BODY"
EXERCISE . TRY TO IDENTIFY
HOW YOU FEEL DIFFERENT

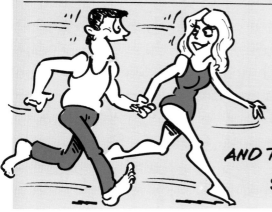

AND IF THERE ARE
TWO OF YOU, WHY NOT
TRY THE EXERCISES
AND THE SHIATSU MASSAGE
STARTING ON PAGE 57 ⇒

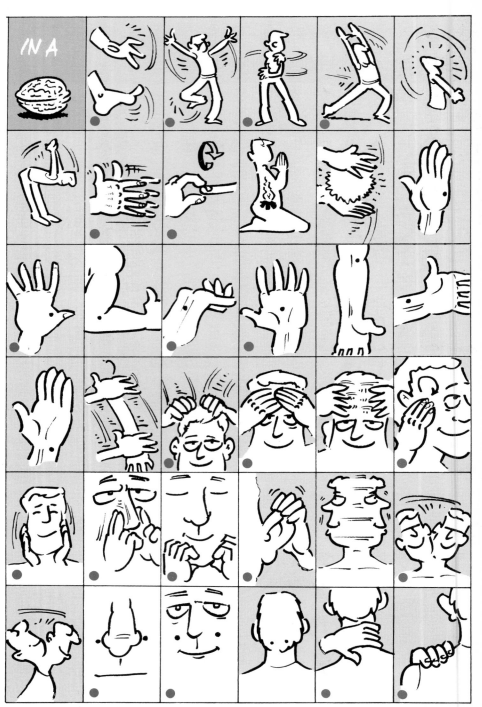

IN A

ALL THE EXERCISES – A FULL 35 MINUTES.

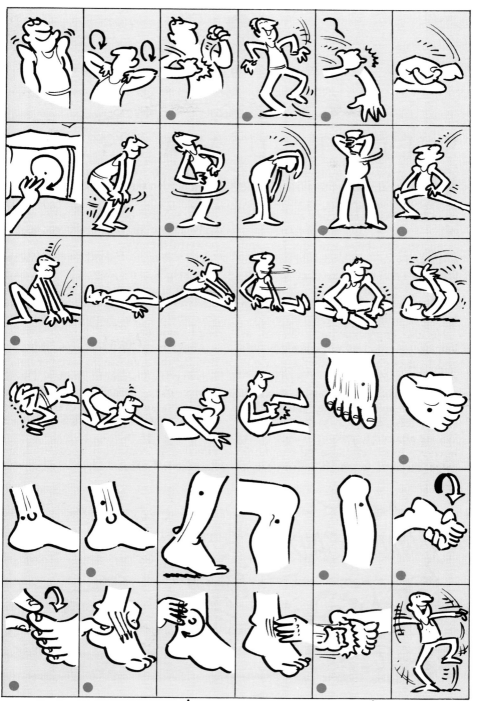

A SHORTENED VERSION (EXERCISES WITH DOTS ●) 20 MINS 54

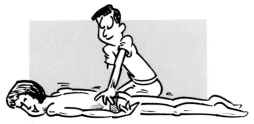

S H I A T S U   M A S S A G E

*S*hiatsu massage is quite simply *Do-In* done by one person to a friend. One person relaxes whilst the other rubs, pounds, presses, stretches and massages.

Shiatsu can be learnt quickly and easily and given to friends and family. In the Orient children were often taught to give their parents and grandparents a regular massage. I have already taught my son to walk up and down my back.

He also enjoys having a shiatsu, as long as it is vigorous and quick! My wife and I often give each other a quick 10 minute shiatsu at the end of the day.

This form of simple shiatsu is excellent to stay relaxed, supple and full of energy. It is a great way to communicate. We are all used to talking to each other, however much can also be communicated through touch. Whether it is a loving touch, healing touch or a comforting touch. In the same way we naturally put our hand to any part of our body where we feel pain. Shiatsu has essentially taken all this and produced a powerful therapy.

The shiatsu practitioner Wataru Ohashi tells an old story set in the Orient of a young newly married woman whose life was made a misery due to the abnormally cruel nature of her husband's mother.

After many years of hardship she decided the only way to save her family was to poison her mother-in-law. On the advice of a herbalist she gave her mother-in-law a potion with the instruction to give a shiatsu after each daily dose for three months to make it more effective. It would then appear that she had died of natural causes. Within two

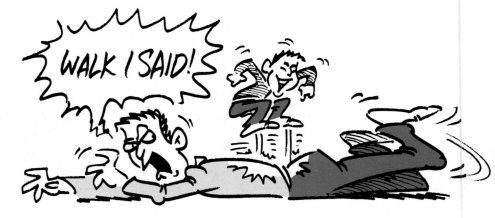

months she began to understand why her mother-in-law behaved as she did. She could feel what her weaknesses and insecurities were. In addition, her mother-in-law became more relaxed and appreciative of her daily shiatsu. She began to grown fond of her daughter-in-law.

Eventually, the young girl realised she was making a terrible mistake and rushed back to the herbalist for an antidote. The wise herbalist simply smiled and admitted that the potion was a harmless flower water. However, he knew that regular shiatsu would help resolve the differences between them.

In addition to family style shiatsu, people also train to become professional Shiatsu practitioners. In Great Britain the Shiatsu Society represents those practitioners who have completed a thorough training and passed the Shiatsu Society assessment.

During a typical shiatsu treatment the patient wears loose cotton clothing.

Shiatsu is normally given on a thin, firm cotton mattress known as a futon, or several layers of blankets placed on the floor. The treatment usually takes an hour.

At the Community Health Foundation, where I work as a shiatsu practitioner, more than 3,000 people have come for a shiatsu each year.

Most come for stress relief, aches and pains, (often in the back and neck) also lack of energy or stress related symptoms such as allergies, skin problems or PMT. Everyone is different, and like may therapists, shiatsu practitioners treat people rather than illnesses. However it is my impression that shiatsu is particularly effective for the symptoms mentioned above, especially if the patient is prepared to make changes in their diet and try exercises between treatments.

Like *Do-In*, shiatsu has to be experienced to be appreciated, and on the following pages you will find a simple shiatsu routine working on the back that you can try with your friends.

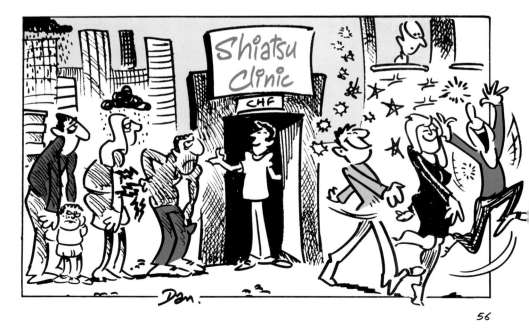

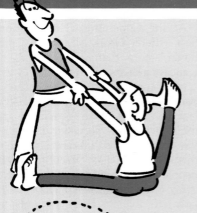

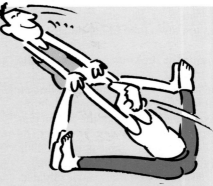

BACKWARDS & FORWARDS X 3 EACH WAY

(STRETCH BUT DON'T STRAIN)

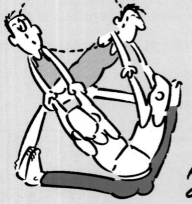

GOOD FOR STRETCHING THE LOWER BACK & INSIDE OF LEGS

MOVE AROUND IN A CIRCLE X 3 EACH WAY

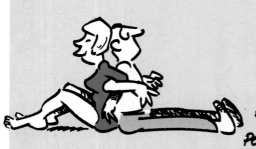

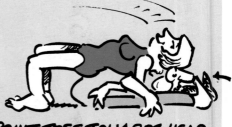

POINT TOES TOWARDS HEAD

GOOD FOR LOWER BACK & CALF MUSCLES X 3 EACH WAY

BACK STRETCHING

2 MIN

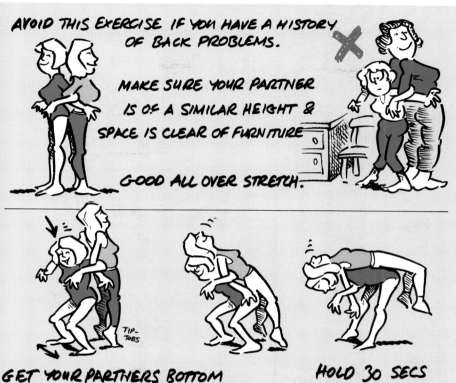

AVOID THIS EXERCISE IF YOU HAVE A HISTORY OF BACK PROBLEMS.

MAKE SURE YOUR PARTNER IS OF A SIMILAR HEIGHT & SPACE IS CLEAR OF FURNITURE

GOOD ALL OVER STRETCH.

TIP-TOES

GET YOUR PARTNERS BOTTOM LEVEL WITH THE SMALL OF YOUR BACK.

HOLD 30 SECS THEN SWOP ROUND

---

1 MIN

LEG STRETCHING

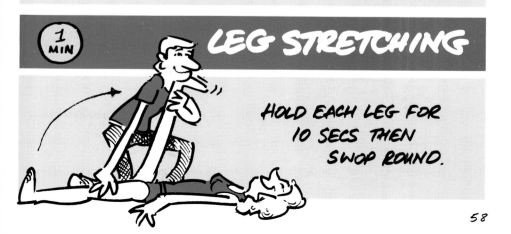

HOLD EACH LEG FOR 10 SECS THEN SWOP ROUND.

POUNDING & BRUSHING

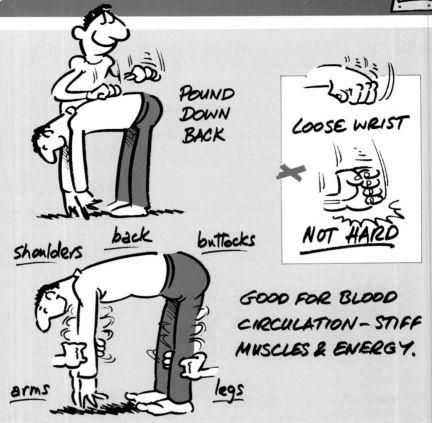

POUND DOWN BACK

LOOSE WRIST

✗ NOT HARD

shoulders   back   buttocks

arms   legs

GOOD FOR BLOOD CIRCULATION – STIFF MUSCLES & ENERGY.

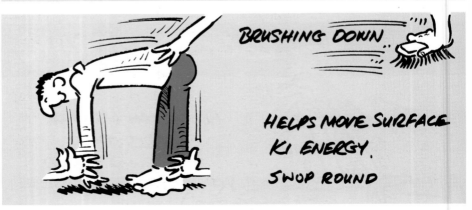

BRUSHING DOWN

HELPS MOVE SURFACE KI ENERGY.

SWOP ROUND

MASSAGE

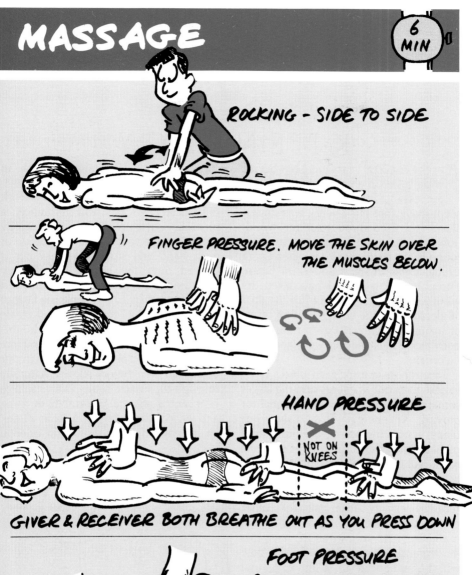

ROCKING - SIDE TO SIDE

FINGER PRESSURE. MOVE THE SKIN OVER THE MUSCLES BELOW.

HAND PRESSURE

NOT ON KNEES

GIVER & RECEIVER BOTH BREATHE OUT AS YOU PRESS DOWN

FOOT PRESSURE
PARTNER LIES FACE DOWN TOES POINTING INWARDS - YOU PUT YOUR HEELS ON THEIR ARCHES IMAGINE GENTLY TREADING GRAPES
THIS IS GOOD FOR MENTAL TENSION & STRESS

60

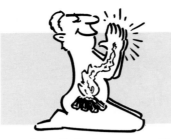

KI ENERGY

For the last 3000 years there has been a wide belief in a living energy that is the essence of all nature. It would seem likely that this energy was understood and used throughout the world, however, the most complete records are found in the East where it is called *Chi* in China, *Prana* in India and *Ki* in Japan. Throughout this book I have used the word *Ki*. *Ki* energy is said to be the flow of electromagnetic energy, and in terms of a human being it flows around the body along invisible pathways known as meridians.

Throughout nature each object takes in and gives out *Ki* energy and the larger something is the greater its potential for moving *Ki* energy. This makes our planet Earth, the Moon, the Sun, other planets and galaxies important in terms of *Ki*. Not only does the earth continually give out energy which we can experience as rising energy, but also receives energy from all the other planets which we experience as descending energy. All around us we have this movement of energy. However this flow will be enhanced in a more natural environment. You will, for example, find you have more energy walking through the countryside than in a large modern indoor shopping centre. A building made of organic materials would obviously be more relaxing and less tiring than one made and furnished with synthetic materials that carry their own static charge. This also applies to clothing.

It is thought that *Ki* energy is both influenced by, and will influence, a physical structure. A good analogy would be of a rough terrain made up of mud, sand and stones. When water is poured onto the terrain it will flow according to the natural valleys, hills and pools. However, after a while the flow of water will change the terrain and create new rivers, pools and islands. In this analogy the land is our body and the water is our *Ki* energy. Therefore in our body our *Ki* energy flows naturally through the easiest route. One is said to be a central channel carrying both rising and descending energy. Michio Kushi, an acknowledged authority on oriental

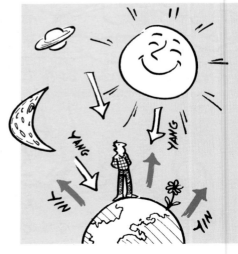

medicine describes how this energy forms seven areas of intense activity like a fast flowing river bubbling around rocks forming whirlpools.

These energy centres are called *Chakras* in India. From these seven chakras flow fourteen large paths of energy known as meridians. Two stay in the torso, six go to the feet and six to the hands. For each meridian one branch goes to the left hand or foot and the other branch to the right hand or foot.

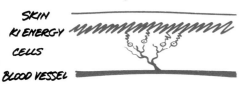

In an interpretation of oriental texts by Michio Kushi, the flow of *Ki* energy mirrors the flow of our blood. In the same way that blood flows through smaller and smaller blood vessels until it finally reaches each cell. *Ki* energy flows through large paths with smaller and smaller branches until they also reach each cell. Each cell is nourished by both blood and *Ki* energy. Blood provides the physical nutrients from our food, water and air such as carbohydrates, proteins, fats, vitamins, minerals and oxygen.

Ki energy represents the unseen, non-physical side of life. It has been described as our soul, spirit, and our connection with nature and consciousness. It is also claimed that our *Ki* energy transports our emotions and ideas to each cell in the same way as our blood transports nutrients. For example; the rush of energy we feel when we have a new exciting idea, the physical strength we have when mentally determined, or the way we feel physically when we are in love, are sensations of *Ki* energy reaching each cell. The feeling of highly charged *Ki* energy is best described as that tingling and alive feeling in every cell of our body.

In Japan there are two words used to describe the condition of *Ki* energy as it flows around the body; *Kyo* and *Jitsu*. When *Ki* energy is deficient or lacking it is described as *kyo* and when there is too much energy, an excess, it is known as *jitsu*. A part of the body that is deficient in energy or *kyo* would typically feel cooler, more hollow and sometimes have a deep pain or bruised feeling when pressed. Alternatively a *jitsu* area will feel more swollen, warmer and tense or stiff when touched. The basic idea is to help *Ki* energy flow better by moving more energy into the weaker *kyo* areas and disperse energy from the tense *jitsu* parts.

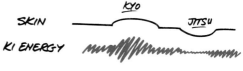

The flow of *Ki* energy can be enhanced by either working on the physical structure through which it flows, (muscles and soft tissue) or directly through the acupressure points. Each point can be stimulated by pressing deeply while breathing out. If a point feels *kyo* it will benefit from long sustained pressure during each slow out-breath. The aim is to try and breathe energy deep into the acupressure point. A more *jitsu* point will benefit from circular massage and more quick short bursts of pressure, also whilst breathing out, to help disperse the energy.

See if you can generate and feel *Ki* energy between your hands by trying the exercise on page 16.

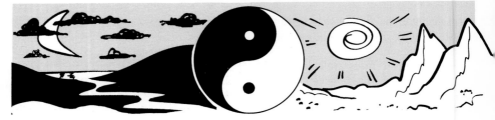

YIN AND YANG

The Yellow Emperor's Classic of Internal Medicine tells us that by 2600 B.C. the Chinese people already had a great interest in the subjective effects of their environment. It describes how they had evolved the concept of a pair of interactive polarities, present throughout nature, which they termed *yin* and *yang*.

The principles of *yin* and *yang* allowed them to make basic connections between their environment (the weather, the seasons, their daily food) and their health and also to describe the essential quality of any phenomena. Nothing was seen to be absolutely *yin* or *yang* but simply more *yin* or *yang* when compared to something else. For example, resting is a more *yin* state that working, which is more *yang*.

In ancient China it was observed that in the morning as the sun comes up people are naturally physically more active and alert; a more *yang* characteristic. In contrast during the afternoon people generally feel more mentally thoughtful, physically passive and sometimes even sleepy which is a more *yin* characteristic.

However, for some people, their day only starts when the moon comes out. The moon creates a more social, creative atmosphere having a more *yin* effect than the sun. It is also interesting to note the difference between a full moon and a new moon. At the time of the full moon

there are more car accidents, violent crimes and disturbances among mentally handicapped patients; all more *yang* effects, whereas a new moon is said to be better for meditation or relaxation; both more *yin* activities.

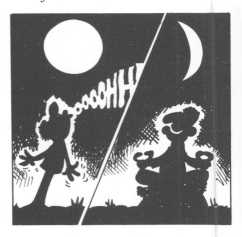

It was also noticed that when someone had a particularly *yang* experience they needed something *yin* to create a kind of balance. For example, if you give guests at a party or customers at a pub, dry, salty snacks which are more *yang* type foods, they tend to crave drinks which are comparitively *yin*, or sweet. The same is true the other way around; lots of fruits, salads and drinks, which are more *yin*, will create a craving for salty, savoury foods.

This cause and effect also applies to the weather. In the Autumn and Winter the air becomes more cold and damp, both *yin* qualities. This creates a need for warming foods like hot porridge, thick soups and stews which are more *yang*, creating balance in the body. Conversely, in the Spring and Summer, as the air becomes warmer and dryer; a more *yang* atmosphere, people then prefer *yin* quality foods that will cool the body, such as fruits, salads and drinks. As everything moves in a cycle of constant change it was thought that *yin* always changed to *yang* and back again. This constant flow can be seen throughout our natural environment. The day (*yang*) changes to night (*yin*). After we rest (*yin*) we go to work (*yang*).

People can also be more *yin* or *yang*. A more *yin* person tends to be relaxed, physically supple, sensitive, creative and imaginative. However, if this person is too *yin* they would become lethargic, slow and depressed. The opposite is true of someone more *yang*. When in balance a *yang* person tends to be alert, quick, physically active, able to concentrate and pay attention to detail. But if the person becomes too *yang* they would become tense, irritable, angry or physically stiff and tight. People often are a mixture of both *yin* and *yang*. However, in the case of a health problem the overriding cause would be attributed to an extreme of one tendency or the other.

With a simple understanding of *yin* and *yang* anyone can tailor their diet, exercise and lifestyle to their own individual needs. For example, if you have a very demanding event next week, between now and then you could eat more *yang* foods and do more *yang* exercises. After this event, *yin* foods and exercises would be ideal to relax and unwind. (See *Healthy Eating* p 65).

In addition, certain aspects of the *Do-In* exercises such as the pounding, rubbing and shaking can be seen as having a more *yang*, energising effect. Whilst the stretches, kneading and breathing techniques have a more relaxing *yin* quality. Practising these techniques will leave the individual feeling more calm and relaxed but also full of energy and vitality.

The philosophy of *yin* and *yang* is open to many interpretations and this book owes a great debt to the work of the Japanese author George Ohsawa. In the 1930s Ohsawa wrote many books on the importance of a good diet to health based on extensive research into the principles of *yin* and *yang*, and natural medicine. The essence of his interpretation is based on the subjective experience of these ancient principles in the individuals daily life.

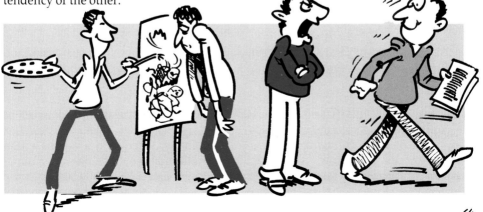

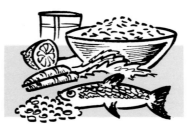

HEALTHY EATING

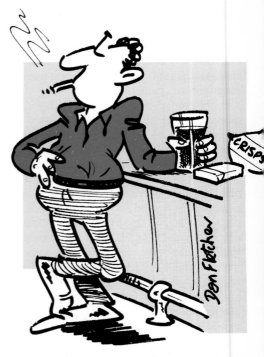

O ne of the great changes in public awareness has been the recognition of the major influence of food on health. The Health Education Authority, the American Government and the World Health Organization, to mention a few, have all published a number of papers confirming the importance of a good diet. Observations have shown that illnesses like heart disease, certain types of cancer, diabetes, arthritis and many other types of what are called degenerative diseases (which is when the body literally degenerates into an unhealthy condition) can be prevented by eating a healthy diet.

The great debate now is – What is a healthy diet? Most people are agreed that a reduction in saturated fats from meat and eggs and all types of dairy foods is a step in the right direction. It is also generally agreed that refined sugar and highly processed foods should be reduced. Instead, more whole grains, fish, beans, fresh fruit and cold pressed vegetable oils are recommended.

In spite of this, claims and counter claims appear regularly and the mass of conflicting research and interpretation can paint a confusing picture. However, in my view, the most sensible approach is to look around the world at those societies that have enjoyed long, healthy lives consistently over many generations and see what their diets have consisted of. Anything less is a risky and unproven experiment.

Much of this work has already been done and synthesized into a set of dietary principles called *Macrobiotics*. Originally, Macrobiotics was based on a traditional Japanese diet after much work by Doctor Sagan Ishizuka in the 1870s. Since then the modern macrobiotic diet has been expanded and now represents foods eaten by most of the world's most healthy societies.

Macrobiotics is based on a diet of grains (whether it is brown rice, barley, porridge, pasta or wholewheat bread) along with fresh vegetables and beans or fish. This is supplemented with fruits, drinks, nuts, seeds, vegetable oils, seasonings, and a few special foods such as tofu, miso, shoyu and sea vegetables.

Each person is a unique individual and follows a different lifestyle and therefore has their own dietary needs. Therefore macrobiotics is based on that flexible set of principles, known as *yin* and *yang* (see page 63) in which certain foods are seen as having a more warming, strengthening and energising effect and are called more *yang*, whereas other foods have a more cooling, relaxing and calming effect, and are seen as being more *yin*.

The principles of *yin* and *yang* can be applied to diet according to our immediate requirements. For exam-ple, if you wanted to do hard physical work outside on a cold day, a thick bean soup, fish casserole or oat porridge, (all more *yang* foods) would help. Obviously fruits, salads and juices, (all more *yin* foods) would not be suitable.

Conversely, if you want to relax and feel good when the weather is hot, eating more light *yin* foods like fresh vegetables, juices or salads would be appropriate.

Application of these principles strengthens our relationship with the planet's natural foods, so that food is eaten not only for its taste but also to enhance physical well-being.

The only way to know whether there is anything to the macrobiotic approach is to do what I did and try it for three months. See how you feel and if you like it keep experimenting. After a year or two you will be surprised how aware you become about food and how well you can make the best choices for your own health.

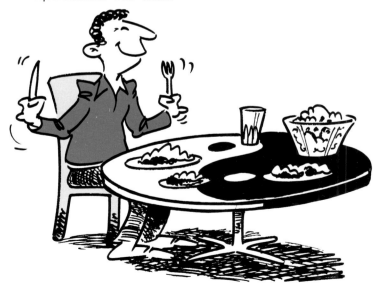

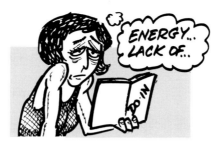

INDEX